Growing Old, Getting Younger:

For Seniors: 5 Minutes Daily Exercises To Keep You Younger And Fit Always.

Debby Anderson

Table Of Contents

The Beginning

First of all, I want to say a big congratulations to you on taking a step toward prioritizing your health and well-being! This book is your guide to maintaining an active and vibrant lifestyle, no matter your age or fitness level.

The fact that you're here, holding this book, shows that you care about your health—and that is the first and most important step.

As one gets of age, staying active becomes more important than ever. The movements you'll find in this book are designed specifically with seniors in mind, offering simple yet effective exercises that can be done in just 5-10 minutes.

These exercises will help you build strength, improve flexibility, boost your energy, and enhance your overall quality of life.

The journey to staying fit at 40 and beyond doesn't require hours in the gym or complex equipment. In fact, research shows that even short bursts of activity can bring incredible benefits to your body and mind. This book is about making fitness approachable, enjoyable, and accessible to everyone.

It's no secret that our bodies change as we age. You might notice a loss of strength, occasional joint stiffness, or decreased energy. These are natural parts of aging, but they don't have to hold you back.

Regular movement—even in small doses—can counteract these effects, helping you stay independent, mobile, and confident.

I also want to implore that you take it slow, steady and consistent. You don't need to transform your life overnight. Success is about consistency, not perfection.

The routines in this book are designed to fit seamlessly into your day. Whether you're a busy grandparent, enjoying retirement, or simply looking for a way to stay active at home, you'll find something here for you.

Each chapter provides step-by-step instructions for short, effective routines that you can do in your living room, at a park, or even while waiting for the kettle to boil. There's no pressure to keep up with anyone else; this is your personal journey to better health.

Think of this book as a roadmap to a more active, joyful future. Whether you're looking to stay strong, reduce joint pain, improve flexibility, or simply feel better in your body, this book offers practical solutions. You don't need expensive equipment, a large space, or prior fitness experience to get started.

Remember, every movement counts. Every time you choose to move instead of sitting still, you're investing in your health and happiness.

As you embark on this journey, I encourage you to keep an open mind and a positive attitude. Celebrate small victories and forgive yourself for the occasional misstep. Health isn't about perfection—it's about showing up for yourself, one day at a time.

Let's start this journey together. As you flip through the pages, you'll learn how to prepare your body, create a safe and effective exercise space, and discover daily routines that will keep you feeling strong and agile. Let's make movement a joyful and lasting part of your life.

Chapter 1
Understanding Your Body

As we grow older, our bodies undergo natural changes. These changes are not barriers but signals guiding us toward what our bodies need to thrive. By understanding these changes, you can adapt your exercise routine to support your health and enjoy an active, fulfilling life.

We are going to explore the most common physical changes people experience after 40, helping you embrace them with knowledge and confidence.

You'll learn how movement can address these shifts and even reverse some of their effects.

Common Physical Changes After 40

One of the major physical changes that occur as one gets older is the decline in muscle mass otherwise known as **Muscle Mass Decline (Sarcopenia)**

What happens starting at your 30s and 40s is that your muscle mass gradually decreases and by 50, you may notice reduced strength and endurance.

As a result of having less muscle in the body, it can affect balance, posture, and the ability to perform everyday activities.

Engaging in strength training and bodyweight exercises at this stage becomes paramount to maintain and even rebuild muscles, boosting your functional fitness.

Another health challenge one may face as a result of old age is **Joint Stiffness and Pain**. Body cartilages can wear down, and joints may lose lubrication, leading to stiffness and discomfort. Conditions like arthritis become more common. Stiffness in these joints can limit your range of motion and make movement less enjoyable.

Gentle, consistent movement would help to increase blood flow to joints, reduce inflammation, and enhance flexibility.

Bone Density Loss is another common health issues encountered by seniors. In this case, bone density naturally decreases with age, particularly after menopause for women. This can increase the risk of fractures which is not supposed to be because strong bones are essential for stability and injury prevention.

Weight-bearing activities, even light ones like walking or chair squats, can slow bone loss and strengthen the skeleton. You should o that often.

Changes in Balance and Coordination: The systems that help us balance—vision, inner ear, and muscle strength—can weaken over time. Poor balance increases the risk of falls, which can have serious consequences for older adults.

Balance-focused exercises, such as standing on one leg or heel-to-toe walking, retrain your body and improve stability.

Another health challenge as a result of aging is **Reduced Cardiovascular Endurance**. What happens here is that the heart and lungs may become less efficient at delivering oxygen to muscles. As a result of this, lower cardiovascular endurance can make it harder to enjoy activities like walking, gardening, or playing with grandkids.

Doing cardiovascular exercises, even low-impact ones like marching in place helps to strengthen the heart and improve stamina.

Physical health is deeply tied to mental and emotional well-being. Movement improves not only your body but also your mood and cognition:

- **Mental clarity:** Regular exercise boosts blood flow to the brain, enhancing memory and focus.
- **Stress relief:** Physical activity reduces cortisol levels and releases endorphins, your body's natural mood boosters.

- **Confidence:** Feeling stronger and more capable in your body translates to greater independence and self-assurance.

By addressing both physical and mental health, exercise becomes a powerful tool for overall well-being.

Recognizing and Respecting Your Limits

As beneficial as exercise is, it's essential to listen to your body. Here are some guidelines for knowing when to push and when to rest:

1. **Pain vs. Discomfort:** Discomfort (like muscle fatigue) is normal and part of building strength. Sharp or persistent pain, however, is a sign to stop and adjust.
2. **Slow Progress is Good Progress:** Don't compare your pace or ability to others. Small, consistent efforts lead to big changes over time.

3. **Rest is Productive:** Your body needs time to recover and rebuild. Alternate between active and rest days to prevent overuse injuries.

Every person's aging journey is different, influenced by factors like genetics, lifestyle, and medical history. Before starting any exercise routine, consider pre-existing conditions, such as arthritis, osteoporosis, or cardiovascular issues and (or) also consult a healthcare provider if you have specific concerns or haven't exercised in a while.

Understanding how your body changes empowers you to care for it better. Movement is one of the simplest and most effective ways to stay ahead of the aging curve.

Remember, aging is not a limitation—it's an opportunity to tune into what your body needs and support it through thoughtful, consistent activity.

Safety First

When it comes to exercise, safety is paramount—especially as we age. Proper preparation ensures that your workouts are effective and enjoyable while minimizing the risk of injury.

Whether you're returning to exercise after a long break or starting for the first time, it is necessary that you make a proper preparation for a safe environment before you begin your exercise. One of the best ways to enhance safety in movements is through Warm ups and Cool downs.

Why Warm-Ups and Cool-Downs Matter

The purpose of warm ups is to gradually increases blood flow to muscles, prepare joints and connective tissues for movement as well as reduce stiffness and the risk of strain.

The role of cool downs on the other hand is to help your heart rate return to normal beat rate, prevent dizziness by gradually redirecting blood flow and to reduce muscle soreness

<u>Warm-Up Routine (3-5 minutes):</u>

March in Place: Slowly lift your knees, swinging your arms naturally.

Gentle Shoulder Rolls: Circle your shoulders forward and backward.

Ankle Circles: Rotate each ankle clockwise and counterclockwise while seated or standing.

<u>Cool-Down Routine (3-5 minutes):</u>

Deep Breathing: Inhale deeply through your nose, hold for a count of three, and exhale slowly through your mouth.

Seated Forward Stretch: Sit on a chair, extend your legs, and gently reach toward your toes.

Neck Stretches: Slowly tilt your head to each side, holding for 10 seconds.

Avoiding Common Mistakes

Even with the best intentions, certain missteps can hinder progress or lead to injury. Things to avoid include skipping warm ups and cool downs exercises, poor or incorrect posture, overexertion and ignoring pain signals.

Jumping straight into exercise can shock your muscles, while skipping the cool-down may leave you feeling sore or lightheaded.

Incorrect posture on the other hand can strain muscles and joints. For instance, avoid locking your knees during standing exercises. Also keep your back straight and avoid hunching during seated exercises.

Pushing too hard can also lead to fatigue or injury. Always prioritize quality over quantity—short, well-done routines are more effective than overdoing it.

Pain is your body's way of telling you something is wrong. If you experience sharp, sudden, or lingering pain, stop and reassess.

Injury Prevention Tips

1. <u>Start Slow</u>: Begin with low-intensity movements and increase gradually as your body adapts.

2. <u>Use Support When Needed</u>: A sturdy chair, wall, or railing can provide stability for balance exercises.

3. <u>Wear Proper Shoes</u>: Supportive, non-slip footwear reduces the risk of falls and provides cushioning for joints.

4. <u>Stay Hydrated</u>: Drink water before, during, and after exercise to maintain energy and prevent muscle cramps.

5. <u>Create a Safe Space</u>: Clear your exercise area of tripping hazards like loose rugs, cords, or clutter.

Remember that before starting a new routine, especially if you have health concerns, it's wise to check in with a healthcare provider. They can provide specific advice based on your medical history.

Conditions Requiring Extra Care:

Osteoporosis: Avoid high-impact or twisting movements.

Heart conditions: Monitor your exertion level and avoid overexertion.

Arthritis: Focus on joint-friendly movements to reduce stiffness without aggravation.

If possible, consider working with a physical therapist or certified fitness trainer familiar with senior fitness. They can customize exercises to suit your needs.

Safety Tips for Common Conditions

1. For arthritis, stick to gentle, low-impact movements like stretching or swimming and avoid prolonged static positions that can stiffen joints.

2. For osteoporosis, always include weight-bearing exercises, such as walking or light resistance training, to strengthen bones. Avoid forward-bending exercises or jerky, high-impact movements.

3. In heart health related issues, opt for low-intensity cardiovascular exercises, such as walking or slow marching. Monitor your heart rate and stop if you feel dizzy or overly fatigued.

Listening to Your Body

Exercise should leave you feeling energized and accomplished—not overly tired or in pain. Sharp or stabbing pain, sudden dizziness, nausea, or shortness of breath and unusual swelling or weakness in a limb are all signs that you should pay attention to during and after your workout. If you notice any of these signs during your exercises, then it is advisable for you to stop.

If in doubt, pause and reassess. It's always better to err on the side of caution.

Safety is not about restricting movement; it's about moving smartly. By following these guidelines, you'll lay a strong foundation for a successful fitness journey. With the right approach, you'll enjoy the benefits of exercise while reducing the risk of setbacks.

Chapter 2
Creating Your Exercise Space

One of the biggest barriers to consistent exercise is the belief that you need a gym membership or expensive equipment to get started.

The truth is, you can create a safe and effective exercise space right at home or wherever you feel comfortable and I will guide you here in setting up a space that encourages movement, accommodates your needs, and makes exercising something to look forward to.

Choosing the Right Space

The key to a great exercise area is accessibility and comfort. Here's what to consider:

1. **Space Requirements:** You don't need a large area—a clear space about 5x5 feet is enough for most exercises You must also ensure that the space is free of clutter to prevent tripping hazards.

2. **Lighting and Ventilation:** Choose a well-lit area to make it easier to see and maintain proper form .Good ventilation ensures you stay comfortable and energized during your workout.

3. **Flooring:** Hardwood, tile, or carpeted floors are fine for most exercises. Use a non-slip mat for added safety during stretches or floor-based movements.

4. **Access to Support:** Nearby walls, chairs, or countertops can provide stability for balance exercises.

You don't also need fancy equipment to get started. The few affordable and versatile items to consider include a chair, resistance bands, light dumbbells (optional), yoga mat or everyday alternative equipment such as using water bottles as weights, a rolled-up towel as a support cushion, or stairs for step-ups.

If however you enjoy fresh air and natural surroundings and you want an outdoor exercise experience, consider moving your routine outside.

You can use the parks or gardens, patio or balcony with walking trails.

Always consider weather conditions, and dress appropriately for outdoor sessions.

Creating a Motivating Environment

The right environment can inspire you to stay consistent. Here are some tips to make your exercise space inviting:

- Keep a favorite photo, plant, or motivational quote nearby to uplift your spirits.
- Play relaxing or energizing music to set the mood.
- Store your equipment in a basket or shelf within easy reach.
- Have a water bottle and towel ready to stay hydrated and comfortable.
- Turn off the TV or silence your phone (unless you're following a workout video).
- Let family members know this is your dedicated time for self-care.

If you're traveling, staying active is still possible with minimal equipment. Pack essential exercise stuff like a resistance band or two (lightweight and compact), a yoga strap or rolled-up scarf for stretching and a printed or digital copy of your favorite routines from this book.

Find a small space in your hotel room or use outdoor areas like parks to keep up your routine.

Part 2: Daily 5-10 Minute Routines

Chapter 3
Morning Wake-Up Routine

The morning is a crucial time for your body. After hours of lying still during sleep, your muscles and joints may feel stiff or sluggish.

Morning exercises work like a gentle alarm clock for your body, waking up your circulatory system, loosening tight areas, and setting the stage for a productive, pain-free day.

These movements are carefully chosen to be low-impact and easy to follow, requiring minimal space or equipment. By committing just 5-10 minutes each morning, you can reduce morning stiffness, boost blood circulation and enhance your mood for a daily positive outlook.

Detailed Morning Routine (5-10 Minutes)

Below is a fully detailed sequence of exercises designed to be safe, effective, and enjoyable. Perform them in order or customize based on your preferences.

1. Seated Spinal Twist (1 Minute)

<u>Purpose:</u>

- Relieves stiffness in the spine and lower back.
- Enhances flexibility in the torso, aiding in daily movements like turning and reaching.

<u>How to Perform:</u>

1. Sit upright on a sturdy chair with feet flat on the ground and knees bent at 90 degrees.
2. Place your right hand on the chair's backrest and your left hand on your right knee.

3. Slowly twist your torso to the right, starting from your lower back, and turn your head to look over your right shoulder.

4. Hold the position for 10-15 seconds while breathing deeply.

5. Slowly return to the center and repeat on the opposite side.

Tips for Success:

- Keep your back straight throughout the twist—avoid slouching or leaning backward.
- Move gently; the goal is a stretch, not a strain.
- If twisting feels uncomfortable, reduce the range of motion by only turning halfway.

2. Neck Rolls (1 Minute)

Purpose:

- Reduces tension in the neck and shoulders.
- Improves mobility, especially beneficial for reducing tech neck.

•

How to Perform:

1. Sit or stand with your back straight and shoulders relaxed.
2. Lower your chin slowly toward your chest.
3. Roll your head gently to the right, letting your ear move toward your shoulder.
4. Continue rolling your head backward, then to the left, completing a semi-circle.
5. Return to the starting position and reverse the direction. Repeat 4-6 times.

Tips for Success:

- Avoid compressing your neck by moving slowly and deliberately.
- Keep your shoulders relaxed and still.

Common Mistake to Avoid:

- Don't roll your head too far backward, as this can compress the cervical spine.

3. Cat-Cow Stretch (2 Minutes)

<u>Purpose:</u>

- Enhances flexibility in the spine and warms up the core.
- Relieves tension in the back, making it an excellent move for those with mild back pain.

<u>How to Perform:</u>

1. Sit on the edge of a chair or stand with hands lightly resting on a counter for support.
2. Inhale deeply, arching your back gently, and lift your chest upward. Let your belly relax as you look slightly upward (Cow Pose).
3. Exhale and round your back, tucking your chin toward your chest and pulling your belly button inward (Cat Pose).

4. Continue to alternate between Cow and Cat poses, matching the movement to your breath. Repeat 5-8 times.

Tips for Success:

- Focus on slow, controlled movements synchronized with your breathing.
- Avoid over-arching your back during the Cow Pose; aim for a gentle curve.
- If standing feels unsteady, perform the movement seated with your hands on your knees.

4. Heel Raises (1 Minute)

Purpose:

- Strengthens calf muscles and promotes circulation in the legs.
- Improves balance and stability for daily activities like walking and climbing stairs.

How to Perform:

1. Stand near a wall or chair for support.

2. Slowly lift both heels off the ground, rising onto your toes.

3. Hold the position for 2-3 seconds, then lower your heels back down.

4. Repeat 10-12 times.

Tips for Success:

- Keep your movements smooth and controlled. Avoid bouncing.

- Engage your core to maintain balance.

- As you build strength, try performing the exercise without holding onto support.

5. Seated Arm Circles (1 Minute)

Purpose:

- Improves shoulder mobility and warms up the arms.

- Encourages better posture by engaging upper back muscles.

<u>**How to Perform:**</u>

1. Sit upright in a chair with feet flat on the ground.
2. Extend your arms out to the sides at shoulder height.
3. Make small circles forward for 10-15 seconds, gradually increasing the size.
4. Reverse direction and perform backward circles for another 10-15 seconds.

<u>**Tips for Success:**</u>

- Keep your shoulders relaxed and avoid shrugging.
- Start with smaller circles if your shoulders feel tight.
- If extending your arms feels tiring, bend your elbows slightly.

6. Standing Side Stretch (1 Minute)

<u>**Purpose:**</u>

- Stretches the sides of the torso and improves posture.
- Encourages better breathing by opening up the ribcage.

How to Perform:

1. Stand with feet shoulder-width apart, arms relaxed at your sides.
2. Raise your right arm overhead and gently bend to the left, feeling a stretch along your right side.
3. Hold the stretch for 10-15 seconds, breathing deeply.
4. Return to the starting position and switch sides.

Tips for Success:

- Avoid leaning forward or backward; keep the stretch lateral.
- Engage your core for stability.

7. Marching in Place (1-2 Minutes)

Purpose:

- Boosts circulation and gently raises heart rate.
- Warms up the lower body and prepares you for the day's activities.

How to Perform:

1. Stand tall with feet hip-width apart and arms at your sides.
2. Lift one knee to waist height while swinging the opposite arm forward.
3. Alternate sides as if marching, keeping a steady rhythm.
4. Continue for 1-2 minutes, gradually increasing your pace if desired.

Tips for Success:

- Land softly on your feet to minimize impact.
- Engage your arms fully to maximize blood flow and energy.

Customizing Your Morning Routine

Feel free to adjust the routine based on your schedule or energy levels. If you don't have much time or you are always busy with work, try to perform only 3-4 exercises for a 5 minutes session.

When you feel energized, try adding repetitions or extend each exercise slightly.

Whenever you feel sudden stiffness or numbness, spend more time on stretches like Cat-Cow or the Seated Spinal Twist.

Doing this routine every morning, you'll likely notice gradual improvements in flexibility, mood, and energy. Over time, these small daily efforts can compound into significant gains in overall well-being.

Chapter 4
Mid-Day Energy Boost

Many people, especially those over 50, find themselves sitting for extended periods during the day—whether it's reading, watching TV, working, or simply relaxing.

Prolonged sitting can lead to stiffness, reduced circulation, and even fatigue. A 5-10 minute mid-day exercise routine serves as a "reset button" for your body, helping you stay active, alert, and mobile throughout the day.

The goal of mid-day movement is not just physical but also mental. Taking a short break to stretch and move can help to combat fatigue because movement increases blood flow and oxygen to the brain, improving energy and focus.

Mid-day energy boosts also help to prevent muscle tightness as regular breaks reduce the stiffness associated with sedentary activities.

Physical mid-day activity triggers the release of endorphins, enhancing your sense of well-being.

What Makes a Great Mid-Day Routine?

A good mid-day exercise routine should:

1. _Be Quick and Simple_: Focus on exercises that require minimal equipment and can be done almost anywhere.
2. _Target Problem Areas_: Address common tension points, such as the back, neck, hips, and shoulders.
3. _Incorporate Movement_: Include gentle cardio to boost circulation without causing fatigue.

Detailed Mid-Day Routine (5-10 Minutes)

Below is a comprehensive set of exercises designed for mid-day rejuvenation. Feel free to modify based on your comfort level.

1. Shoulder Rolls (1 Minute)

Purpose:

- Relieves tension in the shoulders and upper back.
- Improves posture, especially after long periods of sitting.

How to Perform:

1. Sit or stand with a straight back and arms relaxed at your sides.
2. Slowly roll your shoulders upward toward your ears, then backward in a circular motion.

3. Complete 5-6 backward rolls, then switch directions and roll forward for another 5-6 repetitions.

Tips for Success:

- Focus on slow, controlled movements.
- Avoid shrugging your shoulders too high; keep the movement smooth.

2. Seated or Standing Hip Marches (2 Minutes)

Purpose:

- Activates hip flexors and improves lower-body circulation.
- Enhances balance and stability.

How to Perform:

1. Sit in a chair or stand near a wall for support.

2. Lift your right knee toward your chest as high as you comfortably can, then lower it back down.

3. Alternate sides, lifting the left knee.

4. Continue marching rhythmically for 1-2 minutes.

5. If standing, try to avoid holding onto support for an added balance challenge.

3. Desk or Counter Push-Ups (1-2 Minutes)

<u>Purpose:</u>

- Strengthens the chest, arms, and shoulders.
- Engages the core and improves posture.

<u>How to Perform:</u>

1. Stand facing a sturdy surface like a desk, table, or countertop.

2. Place your hands shoulder-width apart on the surface.

3. Step back so your body forms a straight line from head to heels.

4. Lower your chest toward the surface by bending your elbows, then push back up.

5. Repeat for 8-10 repetitions.

Tips for Success:

- Keep your core engaged to avoid sagging hips.

- Breathe steadily: inhale as you lower and exhale as you push up.

- For less intensity, reduce the distance between you and the surface.

4. Seated Side Twists with Resistance Band (Optional, 2 Minutes)

Purpose:

- Strengthens the core and improves spinal mobility.

- Enhances rotational flexibility for daily tasks like turning or reaching.

How to Perform:

1. Sit upright in a chair with feet flat on the floor.

2. Hold a resistance band or a towel between your hands.

3. Extend your arms in front of you at shoulder height.

4. Slowly twist your torso to the right, keeping your arms extended.

5. Return to center and repeat on the left side.

6. Perform 8-10 twists on each side.

Tips for Success:

- Keep your hips stable and let the movement come from your torso.
- Avoid leaning forward or backward.

5. Standing Side Leg Lifts (1 Minute)

Purpose:

- Strengthens the hips and outer thighs.
- Improves balance and stability.

How to Perform:

1. Stand next to a wall or chair for support.
2. Lift your right leg out to the side, keeping it straight and your toes pointed forward.
3. Hold for 1-2 seconds, then slowly lower.
4. Repeat 8-10 times on each leg.

Tips for Success:

- Keep your torso upright and avoid leaning to the side.
- Engage your core for stability.

6. Seated Chest Opener Stretch (1 Minute)

Purpose:

- Stretches the chest and shoulders, counteracting the effects of sitting.
- Encourages deep breathing for relaxation.

How to Perform:

1. Sit on a chair with your feet flat on the floor.
2. Clasp your hands behind your back (or hold the edges of the chair).
3. Straighten your arms and gently lift your chest upward, pulling your shoulders back.
4. Hold for 10-15 seconds, breathing deeply.
5. If clasping your hands feels uncomfortable, place them on your hips and push your elbows backward.

7. Gentle Marching with Arm Swings (2 Minutes)

Purpose:

- Combines light cardio with upper-body mobility.
- Boosts energy and circulation.

<u>**How to Perform:**</u>

1. Stand tall with feet hip-width apart.

2. Begin marching in place, lifting your knees as high as comfortable.

3. Add arm swings, moving your arms forward and back in rhythm with your steps.

4. Continue for 1-2 minutes at a steady pace.

<u>**Tips for Success:**</u>

- Keep your movements light and rhythmic.

- Adjust the pace to match your comfort level.

-

This mid-day routine is versatile and adaptable. You can perform it all at once by doing a full sequence for a comprehensive 10 minutes session or you can do them in small breaks, spreading the exercises throughout the day, completing 1-2 movements every hour or so.

Common Challenges and Solutions One Might Face

1. **"I Don't Have Time"**: Integrate movements into existing activities. For example, perform leg lifts while brushing your teeth or shoulder rolls while waiting for coffee.

2. **"I Feel Stiff"**: Start with smaller, gentler movements and gradually increase your range of motion.

3. **"I Forget to Move"**: Set a timer or reminder to get up and stretch every 60 minutes.

Chapter 5
Evening Wind-Down Exercises

After a long day, your body and mind may feel tense or fatigued. Evening exercises are designed to gently release built-up tension, calm your nervous system, and prepare your body for restful, restorative sleep. These movements are slow and mindful, focusing on relaxation, flexibility, and light stretching.

Evening exercises can help relieve tension by easing tightness in muscles, especially in the back, neck, and shoulders, enhance flexibility by improving range of motion after a day of activity or prolonged sitting and also help to promote relaxation and sleep quality.

How to Create a Relaxing Atmosphere

Set up a calming environment for your evening exercises:

1. Choose a Quiet Space: Minimize distractions by selecting a quiet, clutter-free area.

2. Dim the Lights: Use soft lighting or candles to create a tranquil atmosphere.

3. Play Soothing Music: Gentle instrumental music can enhance relaxation.

4. Have a Mat or Comfortable Surface: Ensure your space is supportive for floor exercises if needed.

5. Wear Loose, Comfortable Clothing: Opt for breathable materials that allow free movement.

Detailed Evening Wind-Down Routine (5-10 Minutes)

This routine focuses on slow, deliberate movements and stretches to calm your body and mind within 5-10 minutes.

1. Seated Forward Fold (2 Minutes)

<u>Purpose:</u>

- Stretches the back, hamstrings, and calves.

- Promotes relaxation by calming the nervous system.

How to Perform:

1. Sit on the floor or a sturdy chair with your feet flat on the ground.
2. If on the floor, extend your legs straight in front of you. If seated, keep your knees bent.
3. Inhale deeply, sitting tall.
4. Exhale and gently fold forward from your hips, reaching your hands toward your feet or shins.
5. Hold the position for 20-30 seconds, breathing deeply. Slowly return to an upright position.

Tips for Success:

- Avoid rounding your back; hinge at the hips instead.
- Use a yoga strap or towel around your feet for added support if your hamstrings are tight.

- Sit on the edge of a pillow or cushion to reduce strain on your lower back.

2. Cat-Cow Stretch (2 Minutes)

<u>Purpose:</u>

- Loosens the spine and relieves back tension.
- Promotes gentle movement to transition from activity to rest.

<u>How to Perform:</u>

1. Start on your hands and knees in a tabletop position.
2. Inhale as you arch your back, lifting your head and tailbone upward (Cow Pose).
3. Exhale as you round your spine, tucking your chin and tailbone inward (Cat Pose).
4. Repeat slowly for 6-8 breaths, focusing on smooth transitions.

<u>**Tips for Success:**</u>

- Move in sync with your breath, letting it guide your pace.
- Avoid over-arching your back to prevent strain.
- If kneeling is uncomfortable, perform this exercise seated in a chair by mimicking the movements with your upper body.

3. Supine Knee-to-Chest Stretch (2 Minutes)

<u>**Purpose:**</u>

- Releases tension in the lower back and hips.
- Gently stretches the glutes and promotes relaxation.

<u>**How to Perform:**</u>

1. Lie on your back with your knees bent and feet flat on the floor.
2. Hug your right knee toward your chest, clasping your hands around your shin.

3. Hold the stretch for 20-30 seconds, breathing deeply.

4. Lower your right leg and repeat with your left knee.

Tips for Success:

- Keep your opposite leg bent or extended, whichever feels more comfortable.
- Avoid pulling too hard; the stretch should feel gentle.
- Place a pillow under your head for neck support if lying flat feels uncomfortable.

4. Reclined Butterfly Pose (2 Minutes)

Purpose:

- Opens the hips and stretches the inner thighs.

- Encourages deep relaxation.

How to Perform:

1. Lie on your back with your knees bent and feet flat on the floor.
2. Bring the soles of your feet together, allowing your knees to fall outward.
3. Rest your arms by your sides or place one hand on your chest and the other on your belly.
4. Hold the pose for 1-2 minutes, breathing deeply.

Tips for Success:

- Support your knees with pillows if the stretch feels too intense.
- Focus on slow, steady breaths to enhance relaxation.

5. Seated Neck Stretch (1 Minute)

Purpose:

- Relieves tension in the neck and shoulders.

- Reduces stress-related tightness.

How to Perform:

1. Sit comfortably in a chair or on the floor.

2. Gently tilt your head to the right, bringing your ear toward your shoulder.

3. Hold for 10-15 seconds, feeling a stretch along the left side of your neck.

4. Slowly return to the center and repeat on the opposite side.

Tips for Success:

- Keep your shoulders relaxed and avoid shrugging.
- Don't force the stretch; move gently.

6. Child's Pose (1-2 Minutes)

Purpose:

- Stretches the lower back, hips, and thighs.
- Promotes relaxation and a sense of calm.

<u>**How to Perform:**</u>

1. Kneel on the floor and sit back on your heels.
2. Lower your torso forward, extending your arms in front of you.
3. Rest your forehead on the mat or a pillow.
4. Hold the pose for 1-2 minutes, breathing deeply.

<u>**Tips for Success:**</u>

- If your hips don't reach your heels, place a cushion under your thighs.
- Keep your arms extended or rest them by your sides.

- Perform the pose seated by leaning forward onto a table or surface for support.

Guided Breathing Exercise (Optional, 2 Minutes)

End your routine with a simple breathing exercise to transition into a state of deep relaxation.

<u>**How to Perform:**</u>

1. Sit or lie in a comfortable position.

2. Inhale deeply through your nose for a count of 4, feeling your belly expand.

3. Hold your breath for a count of 4.

4. Exhale slowly through your mouth for a count of 6.

5. Repeat for 4-6 breaths, focusing on the rhythm and calmness of each cycle.

Tips for Long-Term Success

1. Make It a Habit: Aim to perform your wind-down routine at the same time each evening, signaling to your body that it's time to relax.

2. Track Your Progress: Use a journal to note how you feel after each session.

3. Combine with Other Relaxation Techniques: Pair the exercises with a cup of herbal tea, a warm bath, or quiet reading time.

Chapter 6
Simple Strength Training for Seniors

As we age, muscle mass naturally declines—a process known as sarcopenia. By the time we reach our 50s and beyond, this loss can lead to reduced strength, mobility issues, and even a higher risk of falls. Strength training is a powerful tool to combat this decline.

Regular strength training offers numerous benefits like helping to maintain and build muscle, strengthening of bones, reducing the risk of osteoporosis, enhancing balance and stability etc.

The good news is that strength training doesn't require heavy weights or long sessions. Simple, consistent exercises using your body weight, light dumbbells, or resistance bands can produce significant results.

What to Know Before Starting Strength Training

a) *Start Small*: Begin with lighter resistance or just your body weight, and gradually increase intensity as your strength improves.

b) *Focus on Form*: Proper technique is essential to prevent injury.

c) *Listen to Your Body*: Avoid overexertion; stop if you feel pain or discomfort.

d) *Consistency*: Aim for 2-3 sessions per week, with at least one day of rest in between.

Equipment You May Need

While most exercises can be done with minimal equipment, having the following can enhance your routine: resistance bands, light dumbbells, chair and mat.

Detailed Strength Training Routine (5-10 Minutes)

This routine targets major muscle groups and is designed to improve functional strength, balance, and mobility.

1. Wall Push-Ups (1-2 Minutes)

Purpose:

- Strengthens the chest, shoulders, and arms.
- Engages the core muscles for stability.

How to Perform:

1. Stand about two feet away from a wall, facing it.
2. Place your hands on the wall at shoulder height and shoulder-width apart.
3. Slowly bend your elbows, bringing your chest closer to the wall.
4. Push back to the starting position.
5. Perform 8-10 repetitions.

<u>**Tips for Success:**</u>

- Keep your body in a straight line from head to heels.
- Avoid locking your elbows when pushing back.
- To make it easier, stand closer to the wall.

2. Seated Leg Extensions (1-2 Minutes)

<u>**Purpose:**</u>

- Strengthens the quadriceps (front thigh muscles).
- Improves knee stability and leg strength.

<u>**How to Perform:**</u>

1. Sit on a sturdy chair with your feet flat on the floor.
2. Straighten your right leg, lifting it parallel to the floor.
3. Hold for 2-3 seconds, then lower it slowly.
4. Repeat with your left leg.
5. Perform 8-10 repetitions per leg.

<u>**Tips for Success:**</u>

- Keep your movements slow and controlled.
- Avoid locking your knee at the top of the movement.

3. Resistance Band Rows (2 Minutes)

<u>**Purpose:**</u>

- Strengthens the upper back and biceps.
- Improves posture by counteracting the effects of prolonged sitting.

<u>**How to Perform:**</u>

1. Sit or stand with a resistance band secured around a sturdy object (like a doorknob).
2. Hold the band with both hands, palms facing each other.
3. Pull the band toward your torso, squeezing your shoulder blades together.

4. Slowly release to the starting position.

5. Perform 8-10 repetitions.

Tips for Success:

- Keep your elbows close to your body during the movement.

- Avoid leaning backward; keep your torso stable.

- Use a lighter band or perform the exercise seated if needed.

4. Chair Squats (2 Minutes)

Purpose:

- Strengthens the legs, hips, and core.

- Mimics the movement of sitting and standing, enhancing functional mobility.

How to Perform:

1. Stand in front of a chair with your feet shoulder-width apart.

2. Lower your body as if sitting down, but stop just before touching the chair.
3. Push through your heels to return to standing.
4. Perform 8-10 repetitions.

Tips for Success:

- Keep your chest lifted and your weight in your heels.

- Avoid letting your knees go past your toes.

- Sit fully on the chair and stand back up if partial squats feel too challenging.

5. Bicep Curls with Dumbbells (1-2 Minutes)

Purpose:

- Strengthens the arms, making everyday tasks like lifting objects easier.

<u>**How to Perform:**</u>

1. Hold a dumbbell in each hand with your arms at your sides, palms facing forward.
2. Slowly bend your elbows, bringing the weights toward your shoulders.
3. Lower back to the starting position.
4. Perform 8-10 repetitions.

<u>**Tips for Success:**</u>

- Keep your elbows close to your body throughout the movement.
- Avoid swinging the weights; use slow, controlled motions.
- Use resistance bands instead of dumbbells for a lighter option.

Cool Down and Stretch (1-2 Minutes)

End your session with gentle stretches to relax the muscles and prevent stiffness.

Example Stretches:

i.   Hamstring Stretch: Sit on a chair, extend one leg forward, and lean slightly forward to feel a stretch in the back of your thigh. Hold for 15-20 seconds on each leg.

ii.   Overhead Reach: Sit or stand and raise one arm overhead, gently leaning to the opposite side to stretch the side of your torso. Hold for 10-15 seconds on each side.

iii.   Wrist Circles: Extend your arms and gently rotate your wrists in both directions to loosen them.

Chapter 7
Balance and Stability Exercises

Balance is an essential skill that allows us to move confidently and safely through daily activities. Unfortunately, balance tends to decline with age due to factors such as reduced muscle strength, changes in vision, and decreased coordination. Poor balance can lead to falls, which are a leading cause of injury among older adults.

Incorporating balance and stability exercises into your routine can help reduce fall risk, enhance mobility and strengthen lower body muscles.

Towards preparing for balance exercises, always ensure to choose a safe space. Always have a sturdy chair, countertop or a wall nearby for support when necessary.

Also make sure to put on a proper footwear with good grip for stability or go bare footed if possible.

Detailed Balance and Stability Routine (5-10 Minutes)

This routine focuses on strengthening the core and lower body while improving coordination and proprioception (your sense of body position).

1. Heel-to-Toe Walk (2 Minutes)

Purpose:

- Improves walking stability and coordination.
- Strengthens the lower leg muscles.

How to Perform:

1. Stand tall with your feet together.
2. Step forward with one foot, placing your heel directly in front of the toes of your other foot.
3. Pause briefly, then step forward with the other foot in the same manner.
4. Continue for 6-8 steps.

<u>**Tips for Success:**</u>

- Look straight ahead rather than down at your feet.
- Use a wall or chair for support if needed.
- Perform the exercise near a countertop for added confidence.

2. Single-Leg Stand (2 Minutes)

<u>**Purpose:**</u>

- Enhances balance and strengthens the core, hips, and legs.

<u>**How to Perform:**</u>

1. Stand next to a chair or countertop for support.
2. Lift one foot a few inches off the ground, keeping your knee slightly bent.
3. Hold the position for 10-15 seconds.
4. Lower your foot and repeat on the other side.

5. Perform 2-3 repetitions per leg.

Tips for Success:

- Focus your gaze on a fixed point for better stability.
- Engage your core muscles to maintain balance.
- Lightly touch the chair or wall for support if needed.

3. Side-to-Side Weight Shift (2 Minutes)

Purpose:

- Improves dynamic balance and coordination.
- Strengthens the hips and legs.

How to Perform:

1. Stand with your feet hip-width apart.
2. Slowly shift your weight to your right foot, lifting your left foot slightly off the ground.
3. Hold for a few seconds, then return to center.

4. Repeat on the other side.

5. Perform 6-8 repetitions per side.

Tips for Success:

- Keep your movements slow and controlled.
- Use a chair for balance if necessary.
- Keep your lifted foot closer to the ground for extra stability.

4. Marching in Place (2 Minutes)

Purpose:

- Enhances dynamic balance and strengthens the hips and legs.

How to Perform:

1. Stand tall with your feet hip-width apart.

2. Lift one knee to hip height, if possible, while maintaining balance.

3. Lower your foot and lift the opposite knee.

4. Continue alternating for 8-10 steps per side.

Tips for Success:

- Swing your arms gently to improve coordination.

- Engage your core to maintain stability.

- Hold onto a chair or countertop if needed.

5. Clock Reach (1-2 Minutes)

<u>Purpose:</u>

- Improves balance and strengthens the core and lower body.

<u>How to Perform:</u>

1. Imagine a clock face on the floor around you.

2. Stand tall in the center with your feet hip-width apart.

3. Reach your right foot forward toward "12 o'clock," then return to center.

4. Repeat the movement to "3 o'clock" and "6 o'clock."

5. Switch to your left foot and reach toward "12," "9," and "6 o'clock."

6. Perform 2-3 repetitions per side.

<u>Tips for Success:</u>

- Keep your movements controlled and deliberate.
- Use a chair or wall for support as you gain confidence.

Cool Down and Stretch (1-2 Minutes)

End your routine with stretches that promote flexibility and relaxation. With regular practice, balance and stability exercises can greatly enhance your confidence, reduce your risk of falls, and improve your overall mobility. These exercises may seem simple, but their impact on your quality of life is profound.

Chapter 8
Core Strength for Everyday Support

Your core muscles—comprising the abdomen, lower back, pelvis, and hips—serve as the central support system for your entire body. These muscles stabilize your spine, allow for smooth movement, and support nearly every physical activity you perform daily, from bending and lifting to walking and standing.

As we age, a weak core can contribute to poor posture, decreased balance and stability, limited mobility and chronic pain Strengthening your core doesn't require intensive workouts. Targeted, gentle exercises can yield significant benefits thereby enhancing your overall quality of your body

Core Strengthening Routine (5-10 Minutes)

This routine targets your core muscles through simple yet effective exercises, many of which can be performed on a chair, mat, or standing.

1. Seated Abdominal Bracing (1-2 Minutes)

<u>Purpose:</u>

- Activates and strengthens the deep abdominal muscles.

<u>How to Perform:</u>

1. Sit upright in a sturdy chair with your feet flat on the floor.
2. Place your hands on your thighs or lightly on your stomach.
3. Inhale deeply, then exhale and gently pull your belly button toward your spine.
4. Hold this contraction for 5-10 seconds, breathing naturally.

5. Relax and repeat for 8-10 repetitions.

Tips for Success:

- Keep your back straight and shoulders relaxed.
- Avoid holding your breath during the exercise.
- If sitting is uncomfortable, perform this exercise lying on your back with your knees bent.

2. Bird Dog (2-3 Minutes)

Purpose:

- Strengthens the lower back, abs, and hips while improving coordination.

How to Perform:

1. Start on all fours on a mat with your hands under your shoulders and knees under your hips.
2. Extend your right arm forward and your left leg back, keeping them parallel to the ground.

3. Hold for 3-5 seconds, then return to the starting position.

4. Repeat on the opposite side.

5. Perform 6-8 repetitions per side.

Tips for Success:

- Keep your spine neutral and avoid arching your back.

- Engage your core throughout the movement for stability.

- If kneeling is uncomfortable, perform the arm and leg extensions while seated on a chair.

3. Standing Side Bends (1-2 Minutes)

Purpose:

- Strengthens the oblique muscles (sides of the abdomen) and improves flexibility.

How to Perform:

1. Stand with your feet hip-width apart and arms at your sides.
2. Slowly bend to your right, sliding your right hand down your thigh.
3. Return to the starting position and repeat on the left side.
4. Perform 8-10 repetitions per side.

Tips for Success:

- Avoid leaning forward or backward; keep the movement purely side-to-side.
- Engage your core to control the motion.
- Perform seated side bends if standing is challenging.

4. Seated Knee Lifts (1-2 Minutes)

Purpose:

- Strengthens the lower abs and hip flexors.

<u>**How to Perform:**</u>

1. Sit on a sturdy chair with your feet flat on the floor.
2. Lift your right knee toward your chest, keeping your back straight.
3. Lower your foot and repeat with the left knee.
4. Perform 8-10 repetitions per leg.

<u>**Tips for Success:**</u>

- Avoid slouching or leaning back; keep your spine upright.
- Use slow, controlled movements for maximum benefit.

- Place your hands on the sides of the chair for added support.

5. Plank on a Table or Wall (1-2 Minutes)

<u>**Purpose:**</u>

- Strengthens the entire core, including the abs, back, and shoulders.

How to Perform:

1. Stand facing a sturdy table or wall.
2. Place your hands on the surface, shoulder-width apart, and step your feet back until your body forms a straight line from head to heels.
3. Hold this position for 10-15 seconds, gradually increasing the duration as you build strength.
4. Rest and repeat 2-3 times.

Tips for Success:

- Keep your core engaged and avoid sagging your hips.
- Maintain a straight line through your spine, avoiding neck strain.
- For a gentler version, stand closer to the table or wall.

Cool Down and Stretch (1-2 Minutes)

End your session with stretches to relax and lengthen the core muscles:

a. Cat-Cow Stretch: Start on all fours, arch your back upward (like a cat) and then gently lower it downward (like a cow). Repeat for 5-6 cycles.

b. Seated Spinal Twist: Sit upright on a chair, place your right hand on your left thigh, and gently twist your torso to the left. Hold for 10-15 seconds and repeat on the other side.

c. Overhead Reach: Sit or stand, interlock your fingers, and stretch your arms overhead, leaning slightly to each side.

Chapter 9
Flexibility and Stretching for Longevity

Flexibility is a key component of fitness that directly impacts mobility, posture, and overall physical comfort. Unfortunately, aging often leads to tighter muscles and reduced range of motion, which can make everyday activities like bending, reaching, and walking more challenging.

Improving and maintaining flexibility can make it easier to move freely and perform daily tasks, alleviate tightness in muscles and joints and also help to prevent injuries.

Stretching is gentle, low-impact, and accessible to all fitness levels, making it an ideal practice for seniors seeking longevity and vitality.

Before you start stretching…

   i.   Warm Up First: Stretching cold muscles can lead to strain. A short warm-up, like marching in place for 2-3 minutes, is recommended.

  ii.   Go Slow: Move into stretches gradually, avoiding sudden or jerky movements.

 iii.   Avoid Pain: A stretch should feel mild and pleasant, not painful.

 iv.   Hold Steady: Avoid bouncing; hold stretches for 10-30 seconds to gain the most benefit.

  v.   Breathe Deeply: Deep, rhythmic breathing helps relax muscles and improves the effectiveness of the stretch.

Flexibility Routine (5-10 Minutes)

This routine targets key muscle groups, ensuring your entire body benefits from improved flexibility.

1. Neck Stretches (1-2 Minutes)

Purpose:

- Relieves tension in the neck and shoulders.

How to Perform:

1. Sit or stand tall with your shoulders relaxed.
2. Tilt your head gently to the right, bringing your ear closer to your shoulder.
3. Hold for 10-15 seconds, then return to the center.
4. Repeat on the left side.
5. Perform 2-3 repetitions per side.

Tips for Success:

- Keep your shoulders down; avoid shrugging them.
- Use slow, controlled movements to avoid strain.

- Place one hand gently on the side of your head for a deeper stretch.

2. Overhead Side Stretch (1-2 Minutes)

Purpose:

- Stretches the sides of your torso and improves spinal flexibility.

How to Perform:

1. Sit or stand with your feet shoulder-width apart.
2. Raise your right arm overhead, keeping it straight.
3. Lean gently to the left, feeling a stretch along your right side.
4. Hold for 10-15 seconds, then return to center.
5. Repeat on the other side. Perform 2 repetitions per side.

Tips for Success:

- Keep your torso upright; avoid twisting.
- Engage your core for balance and support.

3. Shoulder Rolls (1-2 Minutes)

<u>Purpose:</u>

- Loosens tension in the shoulders and improves posture.

<u>How to Perform:</u>

1. Sit or stand tall with your arms relaxed at your sides.
2. Roll your shoulders slowly backward in a circular motion.
3. Perform 8-10 backward rolls, then switch to forward rolls.

<u>Tips for Success:</u>

- Focus on making large, smooth circles.
- Avoid hunching your shoulders during the movement.

4. Seated Forward Fold (2 Minutes)

<u>Purpose:</u>

- Stretches the hamstrings, lower back, and calves.

<u>How to Perform:</u>

1. Sit on a sturdy chair with your feet flat on the floor.
2. Extend one leg straight in front of you, keeping your heel on the ground.
3. Hinge forward at the hips, reaching toward your toes.
4. Hold for 10-15 seconds, then switch legs.
5. Perform 2-3 repetitions per leg.

<u>Tips for Success:</u>

- Keep your back straight; avoid rounding your shoulders.
- Only go as far as is comfortable without pain.

- Use a towel or band to loop around your foot for assistance.

5. Cat-Cow Stretch (2 Minutes)

<u>Purpose:</u>

- Improves spinal flexibility and relieves tension in the back.

<u>How to Perform:</u>

1. Start on all fours with your hands under your shoulders and knees under your hips.
2. Inhale and arch your back, lifting your head and tailbone toward the ceiling (Cow Pose).
3. Exhale and round your spine, tucking your chin toward your chest (Cat Pose).
4. Repeat the sequence for 5-6 slow breaths.

<u>Tips for Success:</u>

- Move slowly and match the movement to your breath.

- Keep your range of motion gentle and comfortable.

- Perform a seated version by rounding and arching your back while sitting on a chair.

Cool Down and Relax (1-2 Minutes)

Finish with deep breathing to relax your body and mind:

1. Sit or lie down in a comfortable position.
2. Close your eyes and take slow, deep breaths, inhaling through your nose and exhaling through your mouth.
3. Focus on relaxing each muscle group as you exhale.

Chapter 10
Relaxation and Mindfulness Practices

Physical fitness and mental well-being go hand in hand. As we age, stress, anxiety, and mental fatigue can take a toll on overall health, leading to issues such as high blood pressure, poor sleep quality, and reduced immune function. Relaxation and mindfulness practices offer a natural and effective way to counter these effects, helping seniors maintain a calm and focused mind while complementing physical exercise routines.

Mindfulness and relaxation techniques are simple, accessible, and require no special equipment, making them ideal for seniors.

How to Begin Mindfulness and Relaxation Practices

I.   **Create a Calm Space:** Choose a quiet area where you can sit or lie down comfortably without distractions.

II. **Use Supportive Tools:** A cushion, chair, or yoga mat can make practices more comfortable.

III. **Set Aside Time:** Dedicate 5-10 minutes daily for relaxation, either at the start or end of your day.

Relaxation and Mindfulness Routine (5-10 Minutes)

This routine introduces simple techniques to relax your body and center your mind.

1. Deep Breathing Exercise (2 Minutes)

<u>Purpose:</u>

- Promotes relaxation by activating the body's parasympathetic nervous system.

<u>How to Perform:</u>

1. Sit comfortably with your back straight, or lie down if preferred.
2. Place one hand on your chest and the other on your belly.

3. Inhale deeply through your nose for a count of four, feeling your belly rise.

4. Hold your breath for a count of four.

5. Exhale slowly through your mouth for a count of six, feeling your belly fall.

6. Repeat for 5-6 breaths.

Tips for Success:

- Focus on making your exhale longer than your inhale.

- Keep your shoulders relaxed throughout the exercise.

- If holding your breath feels uncomfortable, skip the pause and focus on smooth, steady breathing.

2. Body Scan Relaxation (3 Minutes)

Purpose:

- Releases tension and brings awareness to different parts of the body.

How to Perform:

1. Sit or lie down in a comfortable position with your eyes closed.
2. Start by focusing on your toes, noticing any sensations or tension.
3. Gradually move your attention up your body—feet, legs, hips, torso, arms, neck, and head.
4. Pause briefly at each body part, consciously relaxing it before moving on.
5. Finish by taking a few deep breaths and gently opening your eyes.

Tips for Success:

- Move slowly and focus on each area without rushing.
- If your mind wanders, gently bring it back to the body part you're focusing on.
- Use a guided audio recording to assist in maintaining focus during the practice.

3. Seated Mindfulness Meditation (3-5 Minutes)

<u>Purpose:</u>

- Cultivates mental clarity and reduces stress.

<u>How to Perform:</u>

1. Sit on a chair with your feet flat on the ground and hands resting on your thighs.
2. Close your eyes or soften your gaze.
3. Focus on your breath as it naturally flows in and out.
4. When thoughts arise, acknowledge them without judgment and return your focus to your breath.
5. Continue for 3-5 minutes.

<u>Tips for Success:</u>

- It's normal for your mind to wander—what matters is gently bringing your focus back.
- Maintain a relaxed but upright posture.

- If focusing on your breath feels difficult, repeat a calming word or phrase, such as "peace" or "relax," with each breath.

4. Gentle Progressive Muscle Relaxation (3 Minutes)

Purpose:

- Relieves physical tension and promotes a sense of calm.

How to Perform:

1. Sit or lie down in a comfortable position.
2. Start with your feet: Inhale, tense the muscles for 3-5 seconds, then exhale and release the tension.
3. Move up your body, repeating the process with your calves, thighs, abdomen, hands, arms, shoulders, and neck.
4. Finish with a deep breath and notice how your body feels more relaxed.

<u>**Tips for Success:**</u>

- Tense the muscles gently, avoiding any discomfort.
- Focus on the sensation of release as you relax each area.

- Skip any areas where tensing feels uncomfortable and focus only on relaxing.

Cool Down: Visualization Exercise (1-2 Minutes)

<u>**Purpose:**</u>

- Uses positive imagery to calm the mind and enhance relaxation.

<u>**How to Perform:**</u>

1. Close your eyes and imagine a peaceful place, such as a beach, forest, or cozy room.
2. Picture yourself there, engaging your senses—feel the warmth of the sun, hear the sound of waves, or smell the fresh air.

3. Spend 1-2 minutes immersing yourself in this scene.

4. Open your eyes and take a deep breath, carrying the sense of peace with you.

Incorporating relaxation and mindfulness practices into your life can transform your mental and physical well-being. These techniques empower you to manage stress, enhance focus, and foster a sense of calm, complementing the physical benefits of your exercise routine.

Chapter 11
Creating Your Personalized Exercise Plan

Consistency is the cornerstone of any successful fitness regimen. While the exercises in this book are designed to be simple and effective, integrating them into your daily routine in a way that aligns with your unique lifestyle and goals is essential. A personalized exercise plan ensures:

a. **Sustainability:** You're more likely to stick with exercises that fit seamlessly into your schedule.

b. **Balanced Fitness:** Incorporates strength, balance, flexibility, and mindfulness for holistic health.

c. **Goal-Oriented Progress:** Focuses on your specific needs, whether it's improving mobility, reducing pain, or boosting energy.

d. **Adaptability:** Adjusts to your fitness level, health conditions, and preferences.

Step 1: Assess Your Current Fitness Level

Before starting, take stock of where you are physically:

1. *Mobility and Balance:*
   - Can you stand on one foot for at least 10 seconds?
   - Do you find it challenging to bend, reach, or twist?

2. *Strength:*
   - How easily can you rise from a chair without using your hands?
   - Do you struggle to carry groceries or lift light objects?

3. *Endurance:*
   - Can you walk briskly for 5-10 minutes without feeling overly tired?

4. *Flexibility:*
   - Can you touch your toes or clasp your hands behind your back?

Write down your observations. These benchmarks will help track your progress and identify areas that need extra focus.

Step 2: Define Your Goals

Set realistic and meaningful goals. Examples include:

- *Short-Term Goals (2-4 weeks):* Improve posture, reduce joint stiffness, or perform exercises regularly.

- *Mid-Term Goals (1-3 months):* Walk longer distances without fatigue, strengthen core muscles, or improve balance.

- *Long-Term Goals (6+ months)***:** Prevent falls, maintain independence, or increase overall energy levels.

Step 3: Select Your Weekly Routine

A balanced plan should include elements of strength, balance, flexibility, and mindfulness. Below is an example schedule:

Day	Focus	Duration	Example Activities
Monday	Strength	10 minutes	Chair squats, wall push-ups, seated bicep curls
Tuesday	Flexibility	10 minutes	Neck stretches, seated forward fold, side stretches
Wednesday	Balance	10 minutes	Single-leg stance, heel-to-toe walk
Thursday	Core	10	Seated

	Strength	minutes	abdominal bracing, bird dog, knee lifts
Friday	Relaxation	10 minutes	Deep breathing, body scan, visualization
Saturday	Combination	10 minutes	Strength + flexibility (light weight training with stretching)
Sunday	Rest or Mindfulness	5-10 minutes	Meditation, progressive muscle relaxation

This schedule is flexible. Adjust days and durations to fit your availability and energy levels.

Step 4: Track Your Progress

Use a journal or chart to log your exercises, duration, and how you feel afterward. Include notes such as:

- "Felt steadier during balance exercises today."
- "Less back pain after core strengthening routine."
- "Improved flexibility in forward folds."

Tracking progress helps you stay motivated and identify areas needing more attention.

Step 5: Modify as Needed

Your exercise plan should evolve based on your progress and changing needs. Adjustments might include:

- Increasing Reps or Duration: As exercises become easier, add more repetitions or extend the duration.
- Trying New Exercises: Explore different activities to keep your routine interesting and challenging.
- Adapting for Comfort: If an exercise feels uncomfortable, modify it or consult a professional for alternatives.

Adopting a Holistic Approach

To maximize the benefits of your personalized plan, consider these complementary lifestyle habits:

- **Stay Hydrated:** Drink plenty of water before and after exercise.
- **Prioritize Nutrition:** Focus on a balanced diet rich in fruits, vegetables, lean protein, and whole grains.
- **Get Adequate Rest:** Sleep is essential for muscle recovery and overall energy.
- **Stay Positive:** Focus on what you can do rather than any limitations.

Sample Daily Plan

Here's how a typical day could look:

Morning: Deep breathing and 5 minutes of balance exercises.

Afternoon: Strength training (10 minutes).

Evening: Flexibility routine followed by a body scan relaxation.

This book has provided tools to empower seniors above 40 to stay active, healthy, and independent through short, effective exercises. By combining strength, balance, flexibility, and mindfulness practices, you can improve your physical and mental well-being, enjoy a higher quality of life, and reduce the risk of age-related issues.

I wish you a healthy grey days as you bask in youthfulness while running through all the exercises in this book!

Appendix

How To Create Exercise Tracking Templates.

To help you stay on track with your personalized exercise plan, here are two types of tracking templates you can use:

1. Weekly Exercise Tracker

This tracker allows you to log the exercises you complete each day. It includes space for tracking duration, intensity, and how you felt after each session.

Day	Exercise Focus	Exercise	Duration	How I Felt	Notes for Improvement
Monday	Strength	Chair squats, wall	10 mins	Energetic, felt stronge	Add 2 more reps

		push-ups		r	next time
Tuesday	Flexibility	Seated forward fold, side stretch	10 mins	Felt more flexible	Stretch deeper on next round
Wednesday	Balance	Single-leg stance, heel-to-toe	10 mins	Steady, improved focus	Add a minute per exercise
Thursday	Core Strength	Abdominal bracing, knee lifts	10 mins	Slightly fatigued	Focus on breathing
Friday	Relaxation	Deep breathi	10 mins	Very relaxed	Increase

		ng, body scan		, calm	duratio n to 12 mins
Saturd ay	Combinati on	Streng th + flexibi lity	10 mins	Challen ging but doable	Stretch more after strength
Sunda y	Mindfulne ss/Rest	Medit ation, progre ssive muscl e relax	10 mins	Rejuve nated, peacefu l	Try visualiz ations next time

2. Monthly Progress Tracker

This tracker helps you evaluate your progress month by month. It focuses on improvements in strength, balance, flexibility, and mental well-being.

Wk No.	Area of Focus	Starting Level	Current Level	Improvements Noted	Next Goal
Wk. 1	Strength (e.g., chair squats)	5 reps	10 reps	Able to do more without rest	Add 5 more reps next month
Wk. 2	Balance (e.g., single-leg stance)	5 seconds	15 seconds	Improved balance, less wobbling	Hold for 30 seconds
Wk. 3	Flexibility (e.g., forward fold)	Unable to touch toes	Fingers almost touch toes	Greater range of motion in hamstrings	Touch toes comfortably
Wk. 4	Mental Well-Being	Moderate stress	Reduced stress	More calm after mindfulne	Practice daily for relaxatio

	(e.g., stress level)			ss sessions	n

Appendix 2

Frequently Asked Questions (FAQs)

Q1: How do I know if I'm doing the exercises correctly?

A: If you experience discomfort or pain during any exercise, stop immediately and reassess your form. Many exercises can be modified to suit your level. If you're unsure about your technique, consider consulting a physical therapist or fitness professional for guidance.

Q2: What should I do if I feel pain during an exercise?

A: Pain is a signal from your body that something is wrong. Stop the exercise and rest. If the pain persists, consult a healthcare provider to ensure you're not exacerbating an injury. Modify exercises to reduce strain, and always focus on controlled movements.

Q3: How can I stay motivated to exercise regularly?

A:

- Set small, achievable goals.
- Reward yourself when you reach milestones, such as a relaxing bath or a favorite treat.
- Consider exercising with a friend or family member for added support and accountability.
- Keep a progress journal to visually track your improvement.

Q4: What if I miss a day of exercise?

A: Missing a day happens to everyone! The key is to get back on track as soon as possible. Don't feel discouraged; it's all about consistency, not perfection. If you miss one day, continue your routine the next.

Q5: How can I adjust my plan if I have a health condition like arthritis or heart disease?

A: It's essential to consult your doctor before starting any exercise routine. They can help you tailor exercises to accommodate your condition. For example, if you have arthritis, you may need to focus on gentle range-of-motion stretches or low-impact activities. If you have heart disease, avoid strenuous exercises and focus on moderate activities like walking and stretching.

Q6: Can I combine this exercise plan with other activities like walking or swimming?

A: Yes! Walking, swimming, or other low-impact exercises can complement your strength, flexibility, and mindfulness routine. Be sure to listen to your body and balance these activities with the exercises in this book.

www.ingramcontent.com/pod-product-compliance
Lightning Source LLC
Chambersburg PA
CBHW071034250726
48653CB00005B/1846